User Guide

for

Medical Terminology Online

to accompany

The Language of Medicine
Seventh Edition

TECHNICAL WRITER

Linda K. Wendling, MA, MFA
Writing/Learning Theory Consultant
Former Faculty, University of Missouri
St. Louis, Missouri

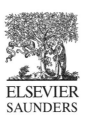

ELSEVIER
SAUNDERS

ELSEVIER
SAUNDERS

The Curtis Center
Independence Square West
Philadelphia, Pennsylvania 19106-3399

MEDICAL TERMINOLOGY ONLINE:
TO ACCOMPANY
THE LANGUAGE OF MEDICINE
Seventh Edition
Copyright © 2004, Elsevier (USA). All rights reserved.

NOTICE

Health care is an ever-changing field. Standard safety precautions
must be followed, but as new research and clinical experience
broaden our knowledge, changes in treatment and drug therapy may
become necessary or appropriate. Readers are advised to check the
most current product information provided by the manufacturer of
each drug to be administered to verify the recommended dose, the
method and duration of administration, and contraindications. It is
the responsibility of the licensed prescriber, relying on experience
and knowledge of the patient, to determine dosages and the best
treatment for each individual patient. Neither the publisher nor the
editor assumes any liability for any injury and/or damage to persons
or property arising from this publication.

ISBN-13: 978-1-4160-0114-0
ISBN-10: 1-4160-0114-X

Evolve® is a registered trademark of Elsevier Inc. in the United States
and/or other jurisdictions

Publishing Director: Andrew Allen
Executive Editor: Jeanne Wilke
Senior Developmental Editor: Billi Sharp
Online Development Team: Jim Twickler, Michael Williams, Christopher Lay, Kristin Korte

Printed in the United States of America

Last digit is the print number: 9 8 7 6 5 4

GETTING STARTED

If your course is being led by an instructor:

1. System

Your instructor will provide information about the system on which your course is being hosted. Evolve® courses can be run on a variety of systems and your instructor will decide which one is right for this course.

2. Username & Password

Your instructor will also provide you with the username and password needed to access the system where this course is located.

3. Login Instructions

If your instructor's course is being hosted on the Evolve Learning System, please go to page 8 for instructions about how to log in. If your course is on a different system, your instructor will provide information about how to log in.

4. Access Code

The first time you access this course, you will need the access code located inside the front cover of this User Guide, regardless of which system is hosting the course. When you are prompted, enter the code exactly as it appears in this guide.

If you plan to take the course on your own:

(**Note:** By taking the course independently, you will not have any instructor to help you with the course. You will have 12 months from the date you are enrolled to complete the course.)

1. System

All independent learners are enrolled in a course hosted on the Evolve Learning System.

2. Self-Enrollment

Please go to page 8 for the instructions about how to self-enroll in the course.

3. Username & Password

If you don't have an existing Evolve account, you will be able to create one during the self-enrollment process.

4. Login Instructions

Please go to page 8 for instructions about how to log in to the Evolve Learning System.

5. Access Code

The first time you access this course, you will need the access code located inside the front cover of this User Guide. When you are prompted, enter the code **exactly** as it appears in this guide.

TECHNICAL REQUIREMENTS

To use an Evolve Online Course, you will need access to a computer that is connected to the Internet and equipped with web browser software that supports frames. For optimal performance, it is recommended that you have speakers and use a high-speed Internet connection. However, slower dial-up modems (56K minimum) are acceptable.

Screen Settings

For best results, the resolution of your computer monitor should be set at a minimum of 800 x 600. The number of colors displayed should be set to "thousands or higher" (High Color or 16 bit) or "millions of colors" (True Color or 24 bit). To set the resolution:

Windows
1. From the **Start** menu, select **Settings** and **Control Panel**.
2. Double-click on the **Display** icon.
3. Click on the **Settings** tab.
4. In the **Screen area** use the slider bar to select **800 by 600 pixels**.
5. In the **Colors** drop down menu, click on the arrow to show more settings.
6. Click on **High Color (16 bit)** or **True Color (24 bit)**.
7. Click on **Apply**.
8. Click on **OK**.
9. You may be asked to verify the setting changes. Click **Yes**.
10. You may be asked to restart your computer to accept the setting changes. Click **Yes**.

Macintosh
1. Select the **Monitors** control panel.
2. Select **800 x 600** (or similar) from the **Resolution** area.
3. Select **Thousands** or **Millions** from the **Color Depth** area.

Web Browsers

Supported web browsers include Microsoft Internet Explorer (IE) version 5.0 or higher and Netscape version 7.1 or higher.

If you use America Online (AOL) for Web access, you will need AOL version 4.0 or higher **and** one of the browsers listed above. Earlier versions of AOL and Internet Explorer will not run the course properly and you will have difficulty accessing many features.

For best results with AOL:
- Connect to the Internet using AOL version 4.0 or higher.
- Open a private chat within AOL. (This allows the AOL client to remain open, without asking if you wish to disconnect while minimized).
- Minimize AOL.
- Launch one of the recommended browsers.

Whichever browser you use, the browser preferences must be set to enable cookies as well as Java/JavaScript, and the cache must be set to reload every time.

Enable Cookies

Browser	Steps
Internet Explorer 5.0 or higher	1. Select **Tools**. 2. Select **Internet Options**. 3. Select **Security** tab. 4. Make sure **Internet** (globe) is highlighted. 5. Select **Custom Level** button. 6. Scroll down the **Security Settings** list. 7. Under **Cookies** heading, make sure Enable is selected. 8. Click **OK**.
Internet Explorer 6.0	1. Select **Tools**. 2. Select **Internet Options**. 3. Select **Privacy** tab. 4. Use the slider (slide down) to **Accept All Cookies**. 5. Click **OK**. **-OR-** 4. Click the **Advanced** button. 5. Click the check box next to **Override Automatic Cookie Handling**. 6. Click the **Accept** radio buttons under **First-party Cookies** and **Third-party Cookies**. 7. Click **OK**.
Netscape 7.1 or higher	1. Select **Edit**. 2. Select **Preferences**. 3. Select **Privacy & Security**. 4. Select **Cookies**. 5. Select **Enable All Cookies**.

Enable Java

Browser	Steps
Internet Explorer (IE) 5.0 and higher	1. Select **Tools -> Internet Options**. 2. Select the **Advanced** tab. 3. Locate **Microsoft VM**. 4. Make sure the boxes are checked for **Java console enabled** and **Java logging enabled**. 5. Click **OK**. 6. Restart your computer if you checked the **Java console enabled** box.
Netscape 7.1 and higher	1. Select **Edit -> Preferences**. 2. Select **Advanced**. 3. Select **Scripts & Plugins**. 4. Make sure the **Navigator** box is checked to **Enable JavaScript**. 5. Click **OK**.

Set Cache to Always Reload a Page

Browser	Steps
Internet Explorer (IE) 5.0 and higher	1. Select **Tools -> Internet Options**. 2. Select the **General** tab. 3. Select **Settings** from within the **Temporary Internet Files** section. 4. Select the radio button for **Every visit to the page**. 5. Click **OK**.
Netscape 7.1 and higher	1. Select **Edit -> Preferences**. 2. Select **Advanced**. 3. Select **Cache**. 4. Select the **Every time I view the page** radio button. 5. Click **OK**.

Plug-Ins

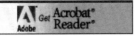

Adobe Acrobat Reader—With the free Acrobat Reader software you can view and print Adobe PDF files. Many Evolve products offer documents in this format, including student and instructor manuals, checklists, and more.

Download at: http://www.adobe.com

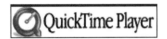

Apple QuickTime—Install this to hear word pronunciations, heart and lung sounds, and many other interesting audio clips within Evolve Online Courses.

Download at: http://www.apple.com

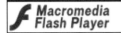

Macromedia Flash Player—This player will enhance your viewing of many Evolve web pages as well as educational short-form to long-form animation within the Evolve Learning System.

Download at: http://www.macromedia.com

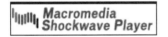

Macromedia Shockwave Player—Shockwave is best for viewing the many interactive learning activities within Evolve Online Courses.

Download at: http://www.macromedia.com

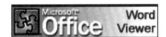

Microsoft Word Viewer—With this viewer, Microsoft Word users can share documents with others who don't have Word software. Users without Word can then open and view Word documents. Many Evolve products have test banks, student and instructor manuals, and other documents available for download and viewing on your local computer.

Download at: http://www.microsoft.com

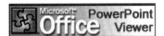

Microsoft PowerPoint Viewer—This viewer makes it possible for you to view PowerPoint presentations even if you don't have PowerPoint software. Many Evolve products have slides available for download and viewing on your local computer.

Download at: http://www.microsoft.com

LOGIN INSTRUCTIONS

IMPORTANT NOTE: These instructions apply only to users whose course is running on the Evolve Learning System. If you are taking an instructor-led course, please ask your instructor which system is hosting your course and where to find applicable instructions. Evolve courses can be run on a variety of systems and your instructor will decide which one is right for a particular course.

1. Go to: http://evolve.elsevier.com/student

2. Enter your username and password in the **Login to My Evolve** area and click the **Login** button.

3. You will be taken to your personalized **My Evolve** page where your course will be listed in the **My Courses** module.

SELF-ENROLLMENT INSTRUCTIONS

IMPORTANT NOTE: These instructions apply only to individuals who will be taking the course on their own. By taking the course independently, you will not have any instructor to help you with the course. You will have 12 months from the date you are enrolled to complete the course.

1. Go to: http://evolve.elsevier.com/Chabner/language

2. Under the **Online Course** heading, click on the **Self-Study Student? Enroll Here** option. This will launch the enrollment wizard for your course.

3. Complete the enrollment wizard. During this process you will create an Evolve username and password. You will also be asked to provide identifying information about yourself and will need to provide the access code from inside the front cover of this guide.

4. Once the wizard has been completed you will be able to log in to your Evolve account and begin your Online Course immediately.

SUPPORT INFORMATION

Technical support is available to customers in the United States and Canada from 7:30 AM to 7:00 PM, Central Time, Monday—Friday by calling, toll-free: **1-800-401-9962**. You can also send an email to <u>evolve-support@elsevier.com</u>.

There is also **24/7 Support Information** available on the Evolve Portal (<u>http://evolve.elsevier.com</u>) including:

- Guided Tours
- Tutorials
- Frequently Asked Questions (FAQ)
- Online Copies of Course User Guides
- And much more!